DASH DIET COOKBOOK

BREAKFAST

---

50 Must-Try Dash Diet Breakfast Recipes

You Will Surely Enjoy!

Anna Cranston

Additionally, the information in the following pages is intended only for informational purposes and should thus be thought of as universal. As befitting its nature, it is presented without assurance regarding its prolonged validity or interim quality. Trademarks that are mentioned are done without written consent and can in no way be considered an endorsement from the trademark holder.

Table of Contents

Introduction

The advantages of Dash Diet for Breakfast are that it consumes less energy and calories than a processed breakfast. Dash Diet for Breakfast promotes the appetite regulation by reducing hunger through a gradual release of sugars, which means you're not going to be peckish until lunchtime. It also avoids the need to count calories because food is recommended in moderation rather than in restriction. To boot, your blood sugar levels will be more stable versus an unhealthy breakfast that spikes and crashes.

The Dash Diet for Breakfast is not a complicated one and to ensure that the benefits are maximized, you need a few basic elements. If you're looking to follow this diet for weight loss, you'll want to eat four or five times per day and be sticking to about 500 calories. If you're going on the Dash Diet for weight loss, but aren't losing weight after several weeks of trying, it may be time to reassess your rigid meal plan. As such, try keeping your meals small and frequent. You can always start by dropping your portions by 10% of your daily intake (for example from 500 calories down to 400). If you're still not losing weight, drop another 10%.

For breakfast you should eat a combination of proteins and healthy carbs. Both help to control your appetite, keep your energy levels up and avoid an early afternoon slump. You need to choose foods that have been reduced or removed from processing to ensure all the fibre, vitamins and minerals remain intact. Your meal plan is going to be largely based on lean proteins like chicken, eggs, fish and pulses, such as beans or lentils. Try your hand at some new vegetarian meals too as vegetables offer a host of nutrients along with fibre and potassium which are vital for weight loss. Aim for around four ounces and remember you can serve vegetables in a number of ways, such as omelettes, frittatas, or even use them in dips.

1.   Easy Veggie Muffins

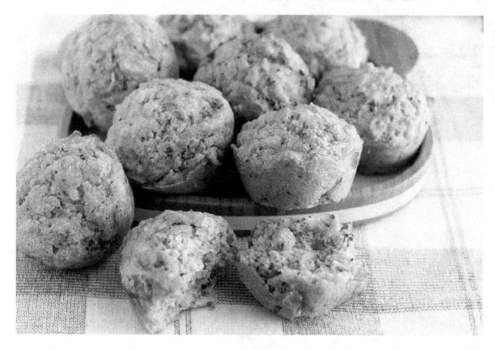

Preparation time: 10 minutes

Cooking time: 40 minutes

Servings: 4

Ingredients:

- ¾ cup cheddar cheese, shredded
- 1 cup green onion, chopped
- 1 cup tomatoes, chopped
- 1 cup broccoli, chopped
- 2 cups non-Fat milk

- 1 cup biscuit ix

- 4 eggs

- Cooking spray

- 1 teaspoon Italian seasoning

- A pinch of black pepper

Directions:

1. Grease a muffin tray with cooking spray and divide broccoli, tomatoes cheese and onions in each muffin cup.

2. In a bowl, combine green onions with milk, biscuit mix, eggs, pepper and Italian seasoning, whisk well and pour into the muffin tray as well.

3. Cook the muffins in the oven at 375 degrees F for 40 minutes, divide them between plates and serve.

Enjoy!

Nutrition (for 100g):

Calories 212, Fat 2, Fiber 3, Carbs 12, Protein 6

2.   Carrot Muffins

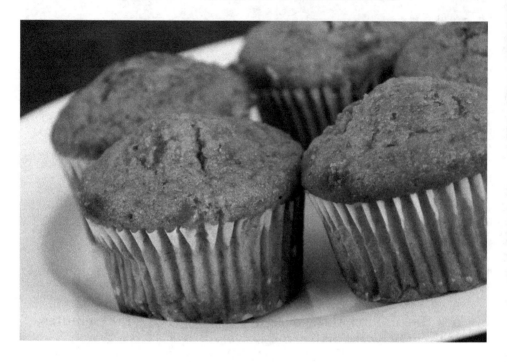

Preparation time: 10 minutes

Cooking time: 30 minutes

Servings: 5

Ingredients:

- 1 and ½ cups whole wheat flour

- ½ cup stevia

- 1 teaspoon baking powder

- ½ teaspoon cinnamon powder

- ½ teaspoon baking soda

- ¼ cup natural apple juice

- ¼ cup olive oil

- 1 egg

- 1 cup fresh cranberries

- 2 carrots, grated

- 2 teaspoons ginger, grated

- ¼ cup pecans, chopped

- Cooking spray

Directions:

1. In a large bowl, combine the flour with the stevia, baking powder, cinnamon and baking soda and stir well.

2. Add apple juice, oil, egg, cranberries, carrots, ginger and pecans and stir really well.

3. Grease a muffin tray with cooking spray, divide the muffin mix, introduce in the oven and cook at 375 degrees F for 30 minutes.

4. Divide the muffins between plates and serve for breakfast.

Enjoy!

Nutrition (for 100g):
Calories 212, Fat 3, Fiber 6, Carbs 14, Protein 6

3.   Pineapple Oatmeal

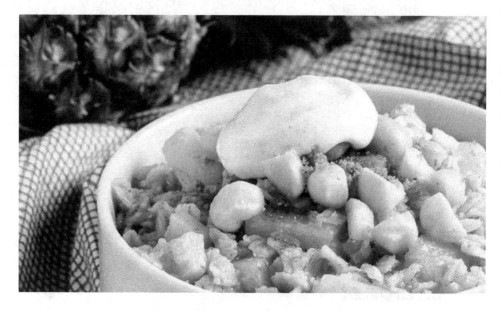

Preparation time: 10 minutes

Cooking time: 25 minutes

Servings: 4

Ingredients:

- 2 cups old-fashioned oats

- 1 cup walnuts, chopped

- 2 cups pineapple, cubed

- 1 tablespoon ginger, grated

- 2 cups non-Fat milk

- 2 eggs

- 2 tablespoons stevia

- 2 teaspoons vanilla extract

Directions:

1. In a bowl, combine the oats with the pineapple, walnuts and ginger, stir and divide into 4 ramekins.

2. In a bowl, combine the milk with the eggs, stevia and vanilla, whisk well and pour over the oats mix.

3. Introduce in the oven and cook at 400 degrees F for 25 minutes.

4. Serve for breakfast.

Enjoy!

Nutrition (for 100g):
Calories 211, Fat 2, Fiber 4, Carbs 14, Protein 6

4. Spinach Muffins

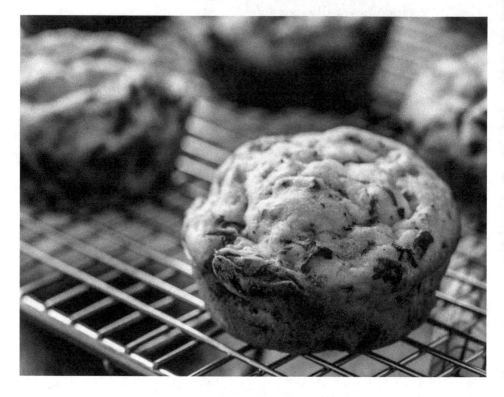

Preparation time: 10 minutes

Cooking time: 30 minutes

Servings: 6

Ingredients:

- 6 eggs

- ½ cup non-Fat milk

- 1 cup low-Fat cheese, crumbled

- 4 ounces spinach

- ½ cup roasted red pepper, chopped

- 2 ounces prosciutto, chopped

- Cooking spray

Directions:

1. In a bowl, combine the eggs with the milk, cheese, spinach, red pepper and prosciutto and whisk well.

2. Grease a muffin tray with cooking spray, divide the muffin mix, introduce in the oven and bake at 350 degrees F for 30 minutes.

3. Divide between plates and serve for breakfast.

Enjoy!

Nutrition (for 100g):
Calories 155, Fat 10, Fiber 1, Carbs 4, Protein 10

5. **Chia Seeds Breakfast Mix**

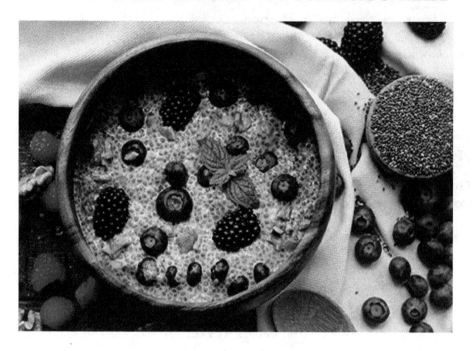

Preparation time: 8 hours

Cooking time: 0 minutes

Servings: 4

Ingredients:

- 2 cups old-fashioned oats

- 4 tablespoons chia seeds

- 4 tablespoons coconut sugar

- 3 cups coconut milk

- 1 teaspoon lemon zest, grated

- 1 cup blueberries

Directions:

1. In a bowl, combine the oats with chia seeds, sugar, milk, lemon zest and blueberries, stir, divide into cups and keep in the fridge for 8 hours.

2. Serve for breakfast.

Enjoy!

Nutrition (for 100g):
Calories 283, Fat 12, Fiber 3, Carbs 13, Protein 8

6. **Breakfast Fruits Bowls**

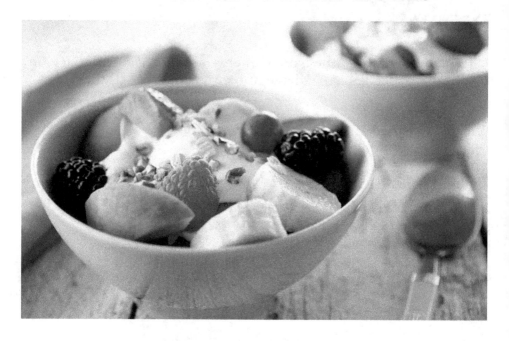

Preparation time: 10 minutes

Cooking time: 0 minutes

Servings: 2

Ingredients:

- 1 cup mango, chopped

- 1 banana, sliced

- 1 cup pineapple, chopped

- 1 cup almond milk

Directions:

1. In a bowl, combine the mango with the banana, pineapple and almond milk, stir, divide into smaller bowls and serve for breakfast.

Enjoy!

Nutrition (for 100g):

Calories 182, Fat 2, Fiber 4, Carbs 12, Protein 6

7. **Pumpkin Breakfast Cookies**

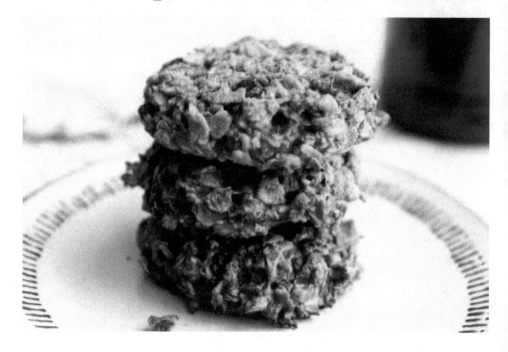

Preparation time: 10 minutes

Cooking time: 25 minutes

Servings: 6

Ingredients:

- 2 cups whole wheat flour

- 1 cup old-fashioned oats

- 1 teaspoon baking soda

- 1 teaspoon pumpkin pie spice

- 15 ounces pumpkin puree

- 1 cup coconut oil, melted

- 1 cup coconut sugar

- 1 egg

- ½ cup pepitas, roasted

- ½ cup cherries, dried

Directions:

1. In a bowl, combine the flour with the oats, baking soda, pumpkin spice, pumpkin puree, oil, sugar, egg, pepitas and cherries, stir well, shape medium cookies out of this mix, arrange them all on a lined baking sheet, introduce in the oven and bake at 350 degrees F for 25 minutes.

2. Serve the cookies for breakfast.

Enjoy!

Nutrition (for 100g):
Calories 281, Fat 12, Fiber 3, Carbs 14, Protein 6

8. Veggie Scramble

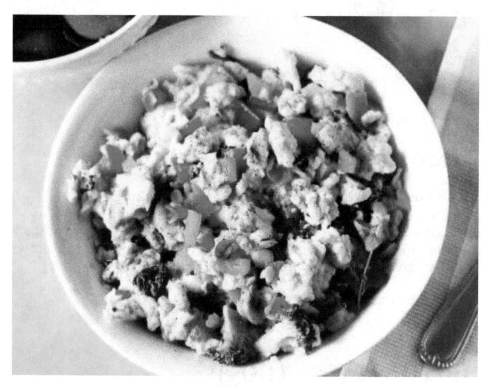

Preparation time: 10 minutes

Cooking time: 2 minutes

Servings: 1

Ingredients:

- 1 egg

- 1 tablespoon water

- ¼ cup broccoli, chopped

- ¼ cup mushrooms, chopped

- A pinch of black pepper

- 1 tablespoon low-Fat mozzarella, shredded 1 tablespoon walnuts, chopped

- Cooking spray

Directions:

1. Grease a ramekin with cooking spray, add the egg, water, pepper, mushrooms and broccoli and whisk well.

2. Introduce in the microwave and cook for 2 minutes.

3. Add mozzarella and walnuts on top and serve for breakfast.

Enjoy!

Nutrition (for 100g):
Calories 211, Fat 2, Fiber 4, Carbs 12, Protein 6

9. **Mushrooms And Turkey Breakfast**

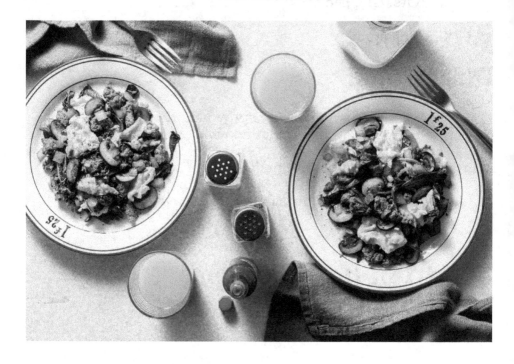

Preparation time: 10 minutes

Cooking time: 1 hour and 5 minutes

Servings: 12

Ingredients:

- 8 ounces whole wheat bread, cubed

- 12 ounces turkey sausage, chopped

- 2 cups Fat-free milk

- 5 ounces low-Fat cheddar, shredded

- 3 eggs

- ½ cup green onions, chopped

- 1 cup mushrooms, chopped

- ½ teaspoon sweet paprika

- A pinch of black pepper

- 2 tablespoons low-Fat parmesan, grated

Directions:

1. Spread bread cubes on a lined baking sheet, introduce in the oven and bake at 400 degrees F for 8 minutes.

2. Meanwhile, heat up a pan over medium-high heat, add turkey sausage, stir and brown for 7 minutes.

3. In a bowl, combine the milk with the cheddar, eggs, parmesan, black pepper and paprika and whisk well.

4. Add mushrooms, sausage, bread cubes and green onions, stir, pour into a baking dish, introduce in the oven and bake at 350

degrees F for 50 minutes.

5. Slice, divide between plates and serve for breakfast.

Enjoy!

Nutrition (for 100g):

Calories 221, Fat 3, Fiber 6, Carbs 12, Protein 6

10. Delicious Omelet

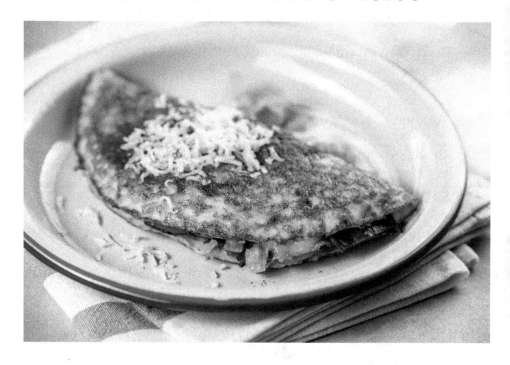

Preparation time: 10 minutes

Cooking time: 6 minutes

Servings: 2

Ingredients:

- 2 eggs
- 2 tablespoons water
- 1 teaspoon olive oil
- ¼ cup low-Fat Mexican cheese, shredded
- ¼ cup chunky salsa

- A pinch of black pepper

Directions:

1. In a bowl, combine the eggs with the water, cheese, salsa and pepper and whisk well.

2. Heat up a pan with the oil over medium-high heat, add the eggs mix, spread into the pan, cook for 3 minutes, flip, cook for 3 more minutes, divide between plates and serve for breakfast.

Enjoy!

Nutrition (for 100g):
Calories 221, Fat 4, Fiber 4, Carbs 13, Protein 7

11. Easy Omelet Waffles

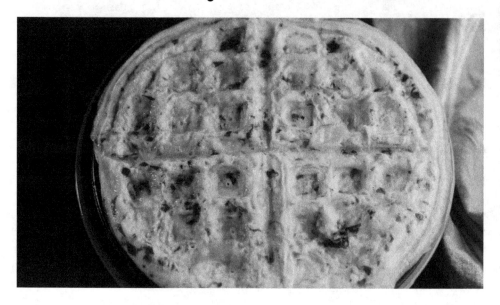

Preparation time: 10 minutes

Cooking time: 5 minutes

Servings: 2

Ingredients:

- 4 eggs

- A pinch of black pepper

- 2 tablespoons ham, chopped

- ¼ cup low-Fat cheddar, shredded

- 2 tablespoons parsley, chopped

- Cooking spray

Directions:

1. In a bowl, combine the eggs with pepper, ham, cheese and parsley and whisk really well.

2. Grease your waffle iron with cooking spray, add the eggs mix, cook for 4-5 minutes, divide the waffles between plates and serve them for breakfast.

Enjoy!

Nutrition (for 100g):
Calories 211, Fat 3, Fiber 6, Carbs 14, Protein 8

12. Jared Omelets

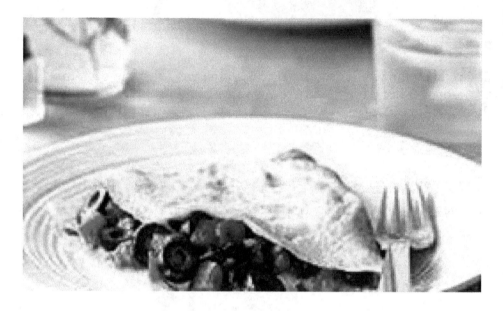

Preparation time: 10 minutes

Cooking time: 6 minutes

Servings: 2

Ingredients:

- Cooking spray

- 2/3 cup low-Fat cheddar, shredded

- 4 eggs

- ½ yellow onion, chopped

- ½ cup ham, chopped

- 1 red bell pepper, chopped

- A pinch of black pepper

30

- 1 tablespoon chives, chopped

Directions:

1. In a bowl, combine the eggs with onion, ham, bell pepper and pepper and whisk well.

2. Grease 2 mason jars with cooking spray, divide the eggs mix, introduce in the oven and bake at 350 degrees F for 6 minutes.

3. Sprinkle the cheese all over and serve for breakfast.

Enjoy!

Nutrition (for 100g):
Calories 221, Fat 3, Fiber 3, Carbs 14, Protein 7

13.   **Mushrooms And Cheese Omelet**

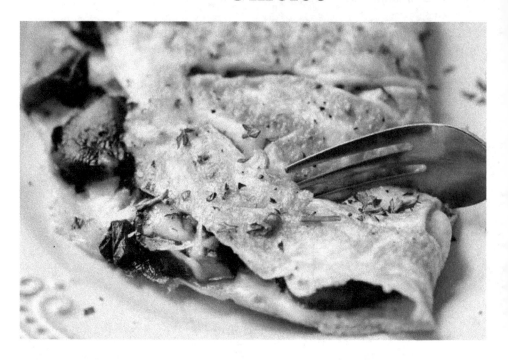

Preparation time: 10 minutes

Cooking time: 15 minutes

Servings: 4

Ingredients:

- 2 tablespoons olive oil

- A pinch of black pepper

- 3 ounces mushrooms, sliced

- 1 cup baby spinach, chopped

- 3 eggs, whisked

- 2 tablespoons low-Fat cheese, grated

- 1 small avocado, peeled, pitted and cubed 1 tablespoons parsley, chopped

Directions:

1. Heat up a pan with the oil over medium-high heat, add mushrooms, stir, cook them for 5 minutes and transfer to a bowl.

2. Heat up the same pan over medium-high heat, add eggs and black pepper, spread into the pan, cook for 7 minutes and transfer to a plate.

3. Spread mushrooms, spinach, avocado and cheese on half of the omelet, fold the other half over this mix, sprinkle parsley on top and serve.

Enjoy!

Nutrition (for 100g):
Calories 199, Fat 3, Fiber 4, Carbs 14, Protein 6

14. **Egg White Breakfast Mix**

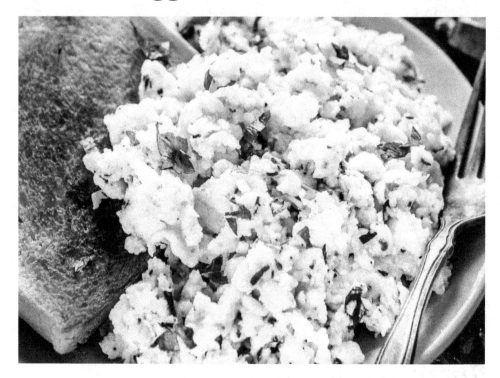

Preparation time: 10 minutes

Cooking time: 10 minutes

Servings: 4

Ingredients:

- 1 yellow onion, chopped

- 3 plum tomatoes, chopped

- 10 ounces spinach, chopped

- A pinch of black pepper

- 2 tablespoons water

- 12 egg whites

- Cooking spray

Directions:

1. In a bowl, combine the egg whites with water and pepper and whisk well.

2. Grease a pan with cooking spray, heat up over medium heat, add ¼ of the egg whites, spread into the pan and cook for 2 minutes.

3. Spoon ¼ of the spinach, tomatoes and onion, fold and add to a plate.

4. Repeat with the rest of the egg whites and veggies and serve for breakfast.

Enjoy!

Nutrition (for 100g):

Calories 235, Fat 4, Fiber 7, Carbs 14, Protein 7

15. Pesto Omelet

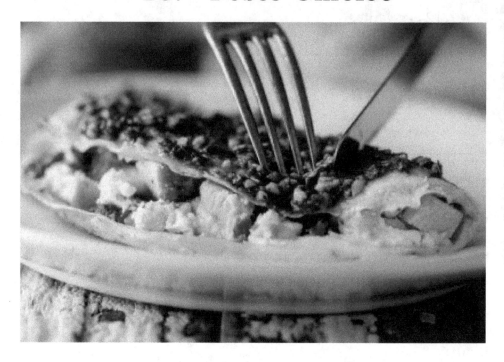

Preparation time: 10 minutes

Cooking time: 6 minutes

Servings: 2

Ingredients:

- 2 teaspoons olive oil

- A handful cherry tomatoes, chopped

- 3 tablespoons pistachio pesto

- A pinch of black pepper

- 4 eggs

Directions:

1. In a bowl, combine the eggs with cherry tomatoes, black pepper and pistachio pesto and whisk well.

2. Heat up a pan with the oil over medium-high heat, add eggs mix, spread into the pan, cook for 3 minutes, flip, cook for 3 minutes more, divide between 2 plates and serve for breakfast.

Enjoy!

Nutrition (for 100g):
Calories 199, Fat 2, Fiber 4, Carbs 14, Protein 7

16. Quinoa Bowls

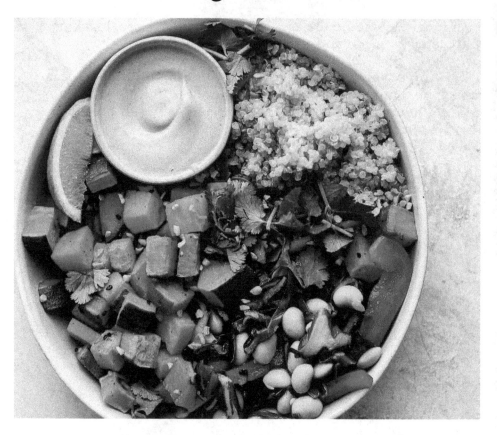

Preparation time: 10 minutes

Cooking time: 20 minutes

Servings: 2

Ingredients:

- 1 peach, sliced

- 1/3 cup quinoa, rinsed

- 2/3 cup low-Fat milk

- ½ teaspoon vanilla extract

- 2 teaspoons brown sugar

- 12 raspberries

- 14 blueberries

Directions:

1. In a small pan, combine the quinoa with the milk, sugar and vanilla, stir, bring to a simmer over medium heat, cover the pan, cook for 20 minutes and flip with a fork.

2. Divide this mix into 2 bowls, top each with raspberries and blueberries and serve for breakfast.

Enjoy!

Nutrition (for 100g):
Calories 177, Fat 2, Fiber 4, Carbs 9, Protein 8

17. Strawberry Sandwich

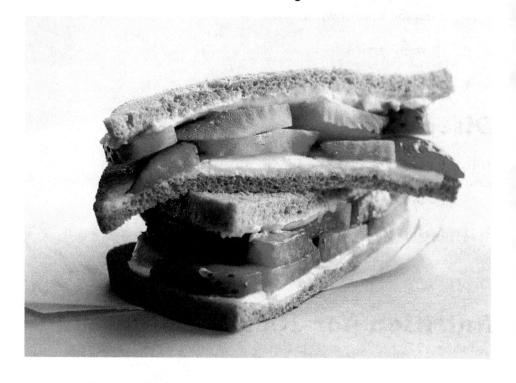

Preparation time: 10 minutes

Cooking time: 0 minutes

Servings: 4

Ingredients:

- 8 ounces low-Fat cream cheese, soft

- 1 tablespoon stevia

- 1 teaspoon lemon zest, grated

- 4 whole wheat English muffins, halved and toasted 2 cups strawberries, sliced

Directions:

1. In your food processor, combine the cream cheese with the stevia and lemon zest and pulse well.

2. Spread 1 tablespoon of this mix on 1 muffin half and top with some of the sliced strawberries.

3. Repeat with the rest of the muffin halves and serve for breakfast.

Enjoy!

Nutrition (for 100g):
Calories 211, Fat 3, Fiber 4, Carbs 8, Protein 4

18. Apple Quinoa Muffins

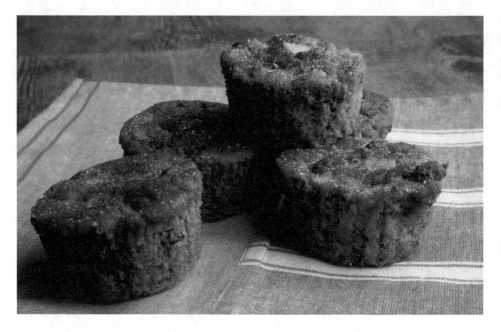

Preparation time: 10 minutes

Cooking time: 35 minutes

Servings: 4

Ingredients:

- ½ cup natural, unsweetened applesauce

- 1 cup banana, peeled and mashed

- 1 cup quinoa

- 2 and ½ cups old-fashioned oats

- ½ cup almond milk

- 2 tablespoons stevia

42

- 1 teaspoon vanilla extract

- 1 cup water

- Cooking spray

- 1 teaspoon cinnamon powder

- 1 apple, cored, peeled and chopped

Directions:

1. Put the water in a small pan, bring to a simmer over medium heat, add quinoa, cook for 15 minutes, fluff with a fork and transfer to a bowl.

2. Add banana, applesauce, oats, almond milk, stevia, vanilla, cinnamon and apple, stir, divide into a muffin pan greases with cooking spray, introduce in the oven and bake at 375 degrees F for 20 minutes.

3. Serve for breakfast.

Enjoy!

Nutrition (for 100g):

Calories 200, Fat 3, Fiber 4, Carbs 14, Protein 7

19. **Amazing Quinoa Hash Browns**

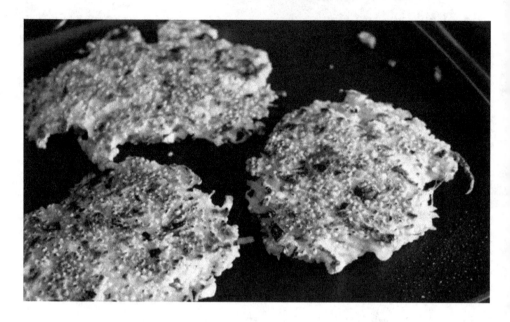

Preparation time: 10 minutes

Cooking time: 25 minutes

Servings: 2

Ingredients:

- 1/3 cup quinoa

- 2/3 cup water

- 1 and ½ cups potato, peeled and grated

- 1 eggs

- A pinch of black pepper

- 1 tablespoon olive oil

- 2 green onions, chopped

Directions:

1. Put the water in a small pan, bring to a simmer over medium heat, add quinoa, stir, cover, cook for 15 minutes and fluff with a fork.

2. IN a bowl, combine the quinoa with potato, egg, green onions and pepper and stir well.

3. Heat up a pan with the oil over medium-high heat, add quinoa hash browns, cook for 5 minutes on each side, divide between 2 plates and serve for breakfast.

Enjoy!

Nutrition (for 100g):
Calories 191, Fat 3, Fiber 8, Carbs 14, Protein 7

20. Quinoa Breakfast Bars

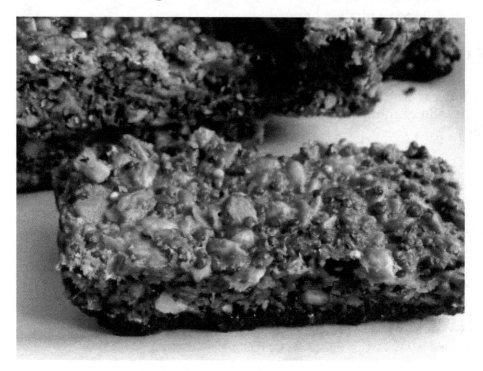

Preparation time: 2 hours

Cooking time: 0 minutes

Servings: 6

Ingredients:

- ½ cup Fat-free peanut butter

- 2 tablespoons coconut sugar

- 1 teaspoon vanilla extract

- ½ teaspoon cinnamon powder

- 1 cup quinoa flakes

- 1/3 cup coconut, flaked

- 2 tablespoons unsweetened chocolate chips

Directions:

1. In a large bowl, combine the peanut butter with sugar, vanilla, cinnamon, quinoa, coconut and chocolate chips, stir well, spread on the bottom of a lined baking sheet, press well, cut in 6 bars, keep in the fridge for 2 hours, divide between plates and serve.

Enjoy!

Nutrition (for 100g):
Calories 182, Fat 4, Fiber 4, Carbs 13, Protein 11

21. Quinoa Quiche

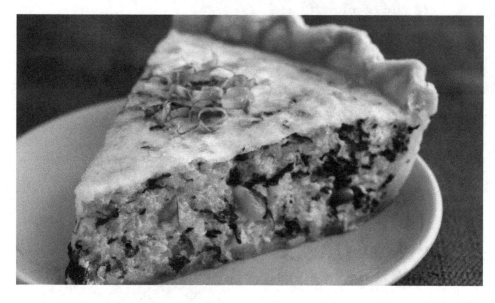

Preparation time: 10 minutes

Cooking time: 45 minutes

Servings: 4

Ingredients:

- 1` cup quinoa, cooked

- 3 ounces spinach, chopped

- 1 cup Fat-free ricotta cheese

- 3 eggs

- 1 and ½ teaspoons garlic powder

- 2/3 cup low-Fat parmesan, grated

Directions:

1. In a bowl, combine the quinoa with the spinach, ricotta, eggs, garlic powder and parmesan, whisk well, pour into a lined pie pan, introduce in the oven and bake at 355 degrees F for 45 minutes.

2. Cool the quiche down, slice and serve for breakfast.

Enjoy!

Nutrition (for 100g):
Calories 201, Fat 2, Fiber 4, Carbs 12, Protein 7

22. **Quinoa Breakfast Parfaits**

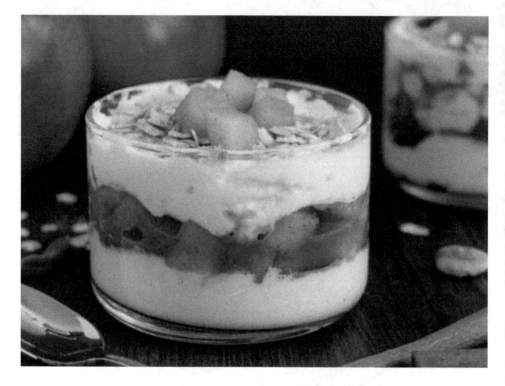

Preparation time: 10 minutes

Cooking time: 20 minutes

Servings: 4

Ingredients:

For the crumble:

- 1 tablespoon coconut oil, melted

- ½ cup rolled oats

- 2 teaspoons coconut sugar

- 1 tablespoon walnuts, chopped

- 1 teaspoon cinnamon powder

For the apple mix:

- 4 apples, cored, peeled and chopped

- 1 teaspoon vanilla extract

- 1 teaspoon cinnamon powder

- 1 tablespoon coconut sugar

- 2 tablespoons water

For the quinoa mix:

- 1 cup quinoa, cooked

- 1 teaspoon cinnamon powder

- 2 cups non Fat yogurt

Directions:

1. In a bowl, combine the coconut oil with the rolled water, 2

teaspoons coconut sugar, walnuts and 1 teaspoon cinnamon, stir, spread on a lined baking sheet, cook at 350 degrees F , bake for 10 minutes and leave aside to cool down.

2. In a small pan, combine the apples with the vanilla, 1 teaspoon cinnamon, 1 tablespoon coconut sugar and the water, stir, cook over medium heat for 10 minutes and take off heat.

3. In a bowl, combine the quinoa with 1 teaspoon cinnamon and 2

cups yogurt and stir.

4. Divide the quinoa mix into bowls, then divide the apple compote and top with the crumble mix.

5. Serve for breakfast.

Enjoy!

Nutrition (for 100g):
Calories 188, Fat 3, Fiber 6, Carbs 12, Protein 7

23. **Breakfast Quinoa Cakes**

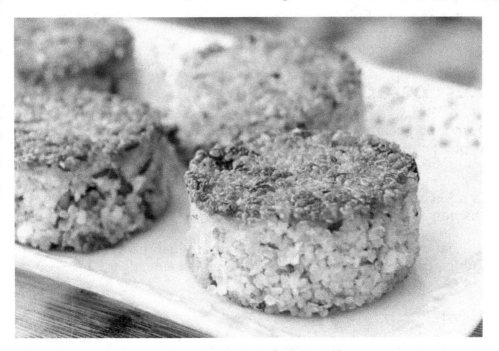

Preparation time: 10 minutes

Cooking time: 30 minutes

Servings: 4

Ingredients:

- 1 cup quinoa

- 2 cups cauliflower, chopped

- 1 and ½ cups chicken stock

- ½ cup low-Fat cheddar, shredded

- ½ cup low-Fat parmesan, grated

- 1 egg

- A pinch of black pepper

- 2 tablespoons canola oil

Directions:

1. In a pot, combine the quinoa with the cauliflower, stock and pepper, stir, bring to a simmer over medium heat and cook for 20 minutes/

2. Add cheddar and the eggs, stir well, shape medium cakes out of this mix and dredge them in the parmesan.

3. Heat up a pan with the oil over medium-high heat, add the quinoa cakes. cook for 4-5 minutes on each side, divide between plates and serve for breakfast.

Enjoy!

Nutrition (for 100g):

Calories 199, Fat 3, Fiber 4, Carbs 8, Carbs 14, Protein 6

24. Easy Quinoa Pancakes

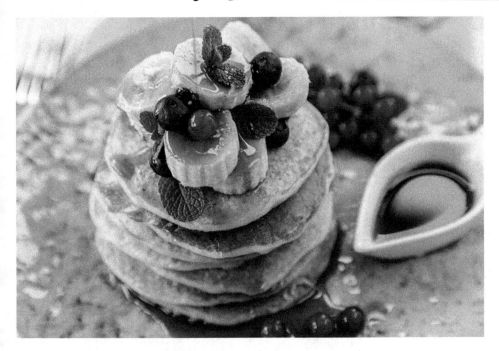

Preparation time: 10 minutes

Cooking time: 6 minutes

Servings: 8

Ingredients:

- ½ cup unsweetened applesauce
- 2 tablespoons coconut sugar
- ½ cup nonFat milk
- 1 tablespoon lemon juice
- 1 teaspoon baking soda

- 1 and ½ cups quinoa flour

Directions:

1. In your food processor, combine the applesauce with the sugar, milk, lemon juice, baking soda and quinoa and pulse well.

2. Heat up a pan over medium heat, spoon some of the pancake batter, spread into the pan, cook for 3 minutes on each side and transfer to a plate.

3. Repeat with the rest of the pancake batter, divide the pancakes between plates and serve for breakfast.

Enjoy!

Nutrition (for 100g):
Calories 188, Fat 3, Fiber 6, Carbs 13, Protein 6

Quinoa And Egg Muffins

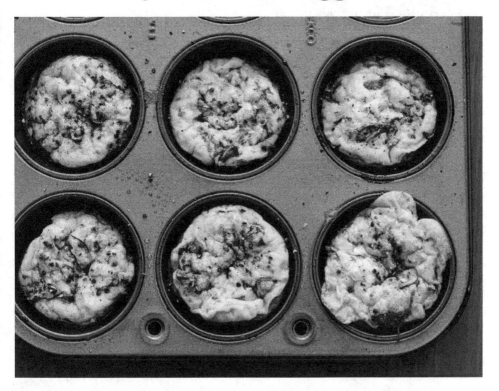

Preparation time: 10 minutes

Cooking time: 30 minutes

Servings: 3

Ingredients:

- 1/3 cup quinoa, cooked

- 1 zucchini, chopped

- 2 eggs

- 4 egg whites

- ½ cup low-Fat feta cheese, shredded

- A pinch of black pepper

- A splash of hot sauce

- Cooking spray

Directions:

1. In a bowl, combine the quinoa with the zucchini, eggs, egg whites, cheese, black pepper and hot sauce, whisk well and divide into 6 muffin cups greased with the cooking spray.

2. Bake the muffins in the oven at 350 degrees F for 30 minutes.

3. Divide the muffins between plates and serve for breakfast.

Enjoy!

Nutrition (for 100g):
Calories 221, Fat 7, Fiber 2, Carbs 13, Protein 14

26. **Apple And Quinoa Breakfast Bake**

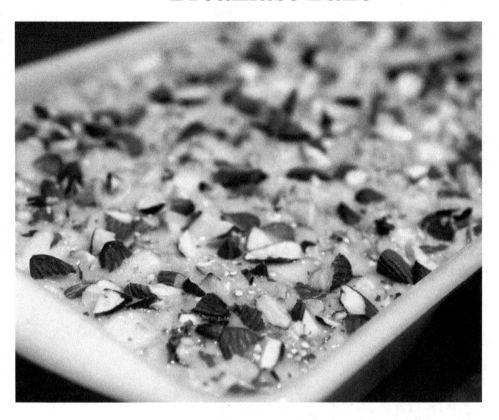

Preparation time: 10 minutes

Cooking time: 10 minutes

Servings: 6

Ingredients:

- 1 cup quinoa, cooked

- ¼ teaspoon olive oil

59

- 2 teaspoons coconut sugar

- 2 apples, cored, peeled and chopped

- 1 teaspoon cinnamon powder

- ½ cup almond milk

Directions:

1. Grease a ramekin with the oil, add quinoa, apples, sugar, cinnamon and almond milk, stir, introduce in the oven, bake at 350 degrees F for 10 minutes, divide into bowls and serve.

Enjoy!

Nutrition (for 100g):

Calories 199, Fat 2, Fiber 7, Carbs 14, Protein 8

27. Quinoa Patties

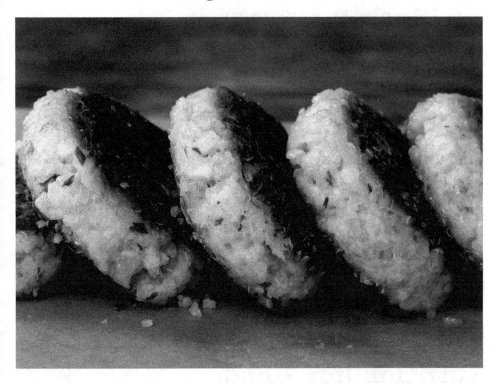

Preparation time: 10 minutes

Cooking time: 20 minutes

Servings: 6

Ingredients:

- 2 and ½ cups quinoa, cooked

- A pinch of black pepper

- 4 eggs, whisked

- 1 yellow onion, chopped

- ¼ cup chives, chopped

- 1/3 cup low-Fat parmesan, grated

- 3 garlic cloves, minced

- 1 cup whole wheat bread crumbs

- 1 tablespoon olive oil

Directions:

1. In a large bowl, combine the quinoa with black pepper, eggs, onion, chives, parmesan, garlic and bread crumbs, stir well and shape medium patties out of this mix.

2. Heat up a pan with the oil over medium-high heat, add quinoa patties, cook them for 10 minutes on each side, divide them between plates and serve for breakfast.

Enjoy!

Nutrition (for 100g):

Calories 201, Fat 3, Fiber 4, Carbs 14, Protein 8

28.   **Peanut Butter Smoothie**

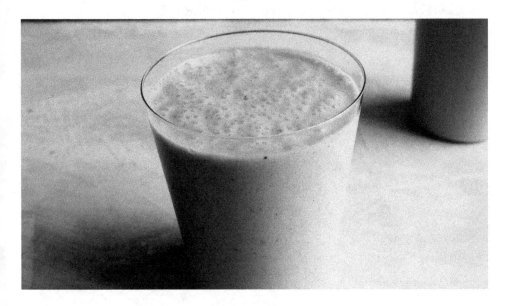

Preparation time: 10 minutes

Cooking time: 0 minutes

Servings: 2

Ingredients:

- 2 tablespoons peanut butter

- 2 cups non-Fat milk

- 2 bananas, peeled and chopped

Directions:

1. In your blender, combine the peanut butter with the milk and bananas, pulse well, divide into 2 glasses and serve.

Enjoy!

Nutrition (for 100g):

Calories176, Fat 4, Fiber 6, Carbs 14, Protein 7

29. Slow Cooked Oatmeal

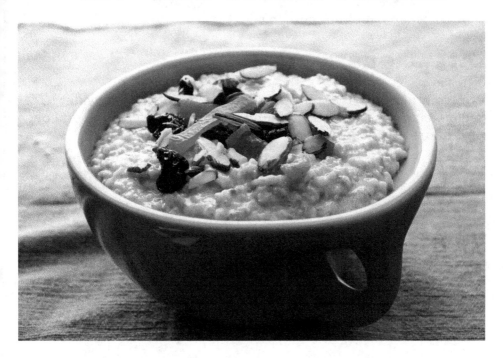

Preparation time: 10 minutes

Cooking time: 8 hours

Servings: 3

Ingredients:

- 4 cups nonFat milk
- 2 cups steel cut pats
- 4 cups water
- 1/3 cup raisins
- 1/3 cup cherries, dried

- 1/3 cup apricots, dried and chopped

- 1 teaspoon cinnamon powder

Directions:

1. In your slow cooker, combine the milk with the oats, water, raisins, cherries, apricots and cinnamon, stir, cover, cook on Low for 8 hours, divide into bowls and serve for breakfast.

Enjoy!

Nutrition (for 100g):
Calories 171, Fat 3, Fiber 6, Carbs 15, Protein 7

30.   **Strawberry And Quinoa Porridge**

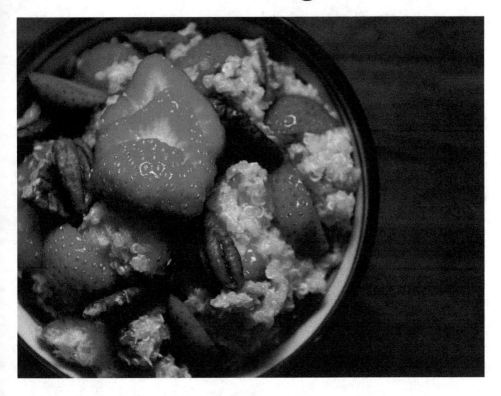

Preparation time: 10 minutes

Cooking time: 15 minutes

Servings: 4

Ingredients:

- 1 cup quinoa

- 2 cups almond milk

- 1 tablespoon coconut sugar

- 1 teaspoon cinnamon powder

- ¼ teaspoon vanilla extract

- 1 cup strawberries, sliced

Directions:

1. In a small pan, combine the quinoa with the milk, stir, bring to a simmer over medium heat and cook for 10 minutes.

2. Add sugar, cinnamon and vanilla, stir, cook for 5 minutes more, divide into bowls, top with strawberries and serve.

Enjoy!

Nutrition (for 100g):

Calories 177, Fat 4, Fiber 7, Carbs 14, Protein 7

31. **Delicious Breakfast Grain Salad**

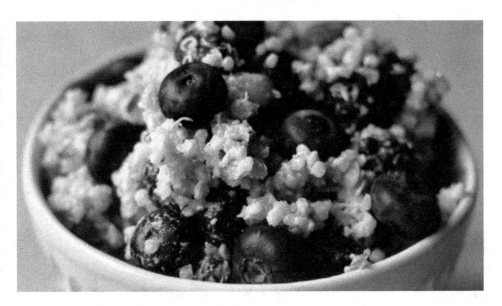

Preparation time: 10 minutes

Cooking time: 10 minutes

Servings: 3

Ingredients:

- 3 cups water

- ¾ cup brown rice

- ¾ cup bulgur

- 1 green apple, cored, peeled and cubed

- 1 red apple, cored, peeled and cubed

- 1 orange, peeled and cut into segments

- 1 cup raisins

- 8 ounces low-Fat yogurt

Directions:

1. Put the water in a pan, bring to a simmer over high heat, add bulgur and rice, stir, cover, reduce heat to medium-low, cook for 10 minutes, spread on a lined baking sheet and leave aside to cool down.

2. In a bowl, combine the grains with the apples, orange, raisins and yogurt, toss and serve for breakfast.

Enjoy!

Nutrition (for 100g):

Calories 181, Fat 3, Fiber 8, Carbs 16, Protein 8

32. Colored Quinoa Salad

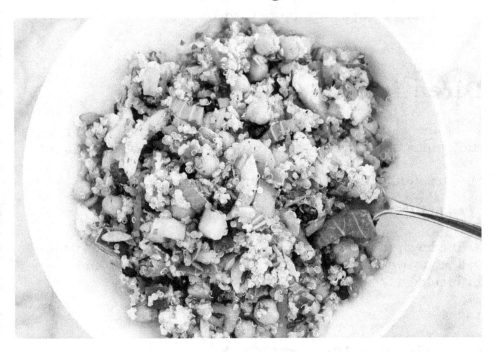

Preparation time: 10 minutes

Cooking time: 20 minutes

Servings: 4

Ingredients:

- 1 cup red quinoa

- 2 cups water

- Juice of 1 lime

- 2 tablespoons stevia

- 2 tablespoons mint, chopped

- 1 and ½ cups blueberries

- 1 and ½ cups strawberries, sliced

- 1 and ½ cups mango, chopped

Directions:

1. Put the water in a pot, bring to a boil over medium-high heat, add quinoa, stir, cover, reduce heat to medium-low, cook for 20

minutes, fluff with a fork and transfer to a salad bowl.

2. Add blueberries, strawberries and mango and toss.

3. In a bowl, combine the stevia with mint and lime juice, whisk well, pour over the salad, toss, divide into small bowls and serve for breakfast.

Enjoy!

Nutrition (for 100g):
Calories 161, Fat 2, Fiber 4, Carbs 10, Protein 8

33. **Moroccan Breakfast Mix**

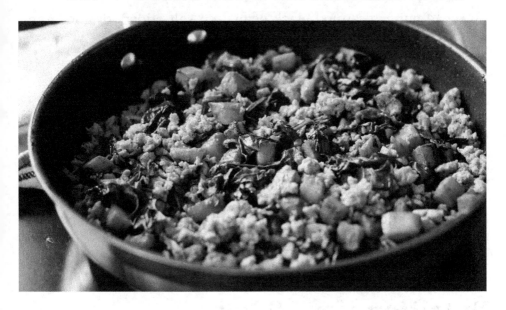

Preparation time: 10 minutes

Cooking time: 20 minutes

Servings: 4

Ingredients:

- 1 cup quinoa

- 1 and ¾ cups water

- 1 tablespoon lime zest, grated

- 3 tablespoons olive oil

- 2 tablespoons lime juice

- 1 teaspoon chili powder

- 1 and ½ teaspoons cumin, ground

- 1 teaspoon coriander, ground

- 14 ounces canned black beans, no-salt-added, drained and rinsed 1 cup cilantro, chopped

- A pinch of black pepper

Directions:

1. Put the water in a pot, bring to a boil over medium heat, add quinoa, lime zest, chili powder, cumin and coriander, cover, cook for 20 minutes, fluff with a fork and transfer to a salad bowl.

2. Add lime juice, olive oil, black beans, cilantro and black pepper, toss and serve for breakfast.

Enjoy!

Nutrition (for 100g):
Calories 201, Fat 3, Fiber 4, Carbs 14, Protein 8

34. Chickpeas Breakfast Salad

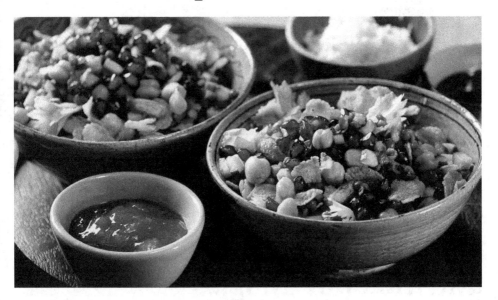

Preparation time: 10 minutes

Cooking time: 0 minutes

Servings: 4

Ingredients:

- 1 tablespoon parsley, chopped

- 1 tablespoon mint, chopped

- 1 tablespoon chives, chopped

- 2 ounces radishes, chopped

- 2 beets, peeled and grated

- 1 apple, cored, peeled and cubed

- 1 teaspoon cumin, ground

- 2 ounces quinoa, cooked

- 3 tablespoons olive oil

- 7 ounces canned chickpeas, no-salt-added, drained and rinsed 7 ounces canned green chilies, chopped

- Juice of 2 lemons

Directions:

1. In a bowl, combine the parsley with the mint, chives, radishes, beets, apple, cumin, quinoa, oil, chickpeas, chilies and lemon juice, toss well, divide into small bowls and serve for breakfast.

Enjoy!

Nutrition (for 100g):
Calories 251, Fat 8, Fiber 8, Carbs 14, Protein 14

35.   **Delicious Blueberry Breakfast Salad**

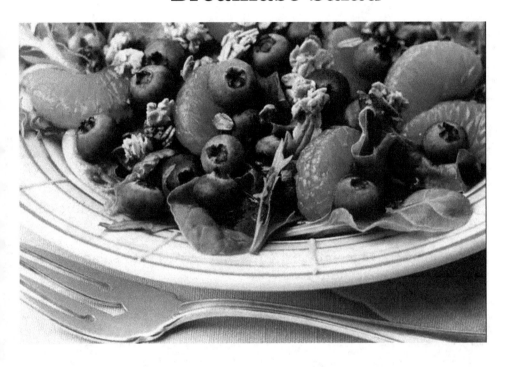

Preparation time: 10 minutes

Cooking time: 0 minutes

Servings: 4

Ingredients:

- 2 pounds salad greens, torn

- 4 cups blueberries

- 3 cups orange, peeled and cut into segments 2 cups granola

- *For the vinaigrette:*

- 1 cup blueberries

- 1 cup olive oil

- 2 tablespoons coconut sugar

- 2 teaspoons shallot, minced

- ½ teaspoon sweet paprika

- A pinch of black pepper

Directions:

1. In your food processor, combine 1 cup blueberries with the oil, sugar, shallot, paprika and black pepper and pulse well.

2. In a salad, bowl, combine 4 cups blueberries with salad greens, granola and oranges and toss.

3. Add the blueberry vinaigrette, toss and serve for breakfast.

Enjoy!

Nutrition (for 100g):
Calories 171, Fat 2, Fiber 4, Carbs 8, Protein 8

36. Kale Breakfast Salad

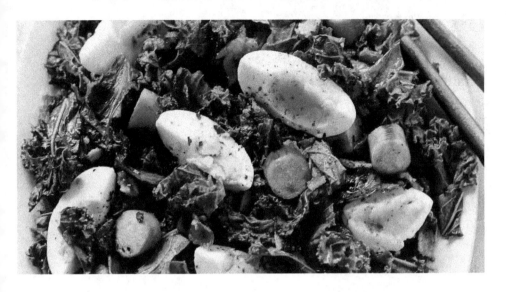

Preparation time: 10 minutes

Cooking time: 0 minutes

Servings: 4

Ingredients:

- 6 cups kale, chopped

- ¼ cup lemon juice

- ½ cup olive oil

- 1 teaspoon mustard

- 1 and ½ cups quinoa, cooked

- 1 and ½ cups cherry tomatoes, halved

- A pinch of black pepper

- 3 tablespoons pine nuts, toasted

Directions:

1. In a large salad bowl, combine the kale with quinoa and cherry tomatoes.

2. Add lemon juice, oil, mustard, black pepper and pine nuts, toss well, divide between plates and serve for breakfast.

Enjoy!

Nutrition (for 100g):
Calories 165, Fat 5, Fiber 7, Carbs 14, Protein 6

37. **Salmon Breakfast Salad**

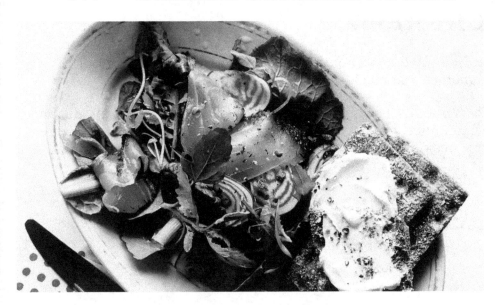

Preparation time: 10 minutes

Cooking time: 0 minutes

Servings: 2

Ingredients:

- 3 tablespoons nonFat yogurt

- 1 teaspoon horseradish sauce

- 1 tablespoon dill, chopped

- 1 teaspoon lemon juice

- 4 ounces smoked salmon, boneless, skinless and torn 3 ounces salad greens

- 2 ounces cherry tomatoes, halved

- 2 ounces black olives, pitted and sliced

Directions:

1. In a salad bowl, combine the salmon with salad greens, tomatoes and black olives.

2. In another bowl, combine the yogurt with horseradish, dill and lemon juice, whisk well, pour over the salad, toss well and serve for breakfast.

Enjoy!

Nutrition (for 100g):
Calories 177, Fat 4, Fiber 7, Carbs 14, Protein 8

38. **Banana And Pear Breakfast Salad**

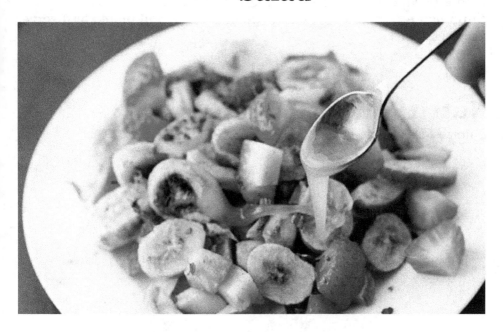

Preparation time: 10 minutes

Cooking time: 0 minutes

Servings: 2

Ingredients:

- 1 banana, peeled and sliced

- 1 Asian pear, cored and cubed

- Juice of ½ lime

- ½ teaspoon cinnamon powder

- 2 ounces pepitas, toasted

Directions:

1. In a bowl, combine the banana with the pear, lime juice, cinnamon and pepitas, toss, divide between small plates and serve for breakfast.

Enjoy!

Nutrition (for 100g):
Calories 188, Fat 2, Fiber 3, Carbs 5, Protein 7

39. Simple Plum And Avocado Salad

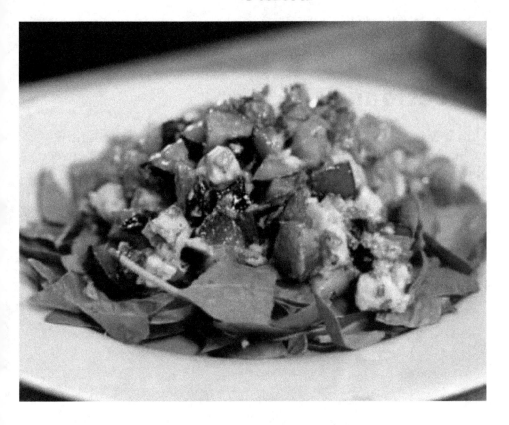

Preparation time: 10 minutes

Cooking time: 0 minutes

Servings: 3

Ingredients:

- 2 avocados, peeled, pitted and cubed

- 4 plums, stones removed and cubed

- 1 cup cilantro, chopped

- 1 garlic clove, minced

- Juice of 1 lemon

- A drizzle of olive oil

- 1 red chili pepper, minced

Directions:

1. In a salad bowl, combine the avocados with plums, cilantro, garlic, lemon juice, oil and chili pepper, toss well, divide between plates and serve for breakfast.

Enjoy!

Nutrition (for 100g):
Calories 212, Fat 2, Fiber 4, Carbs 14, Protein 11

40. Cherries Oatmeal

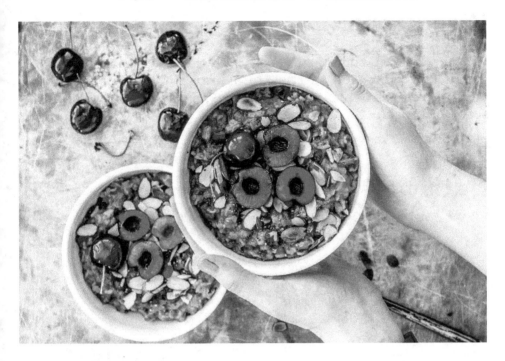

Preparation time: 10 minutes

Cooking time: 15 minutes

Servings: 6

Ingredients:

- 2 cups old-fashioned oats

- 6 cups water

- 1 cup almond milk

- 1 teaspoon cinnamon powder

- 1 teaspoon vanilla extract

- 2 cups cherries, pitted and sliced

Directions:

1. In a small pot, combine the oats with the water, milk, cinnamon, vanilla and cherries, toss, bring to a simmer over medium-high heat, cook for 15 minutes, divide into bowls and serve for breakfast.

Enjoy!

Nutrition (for 100g):

Calories 180, Fat 4, Fiber 4, Carbs 9, Protein 7

41. **Orange And Apricots Oatmeal**

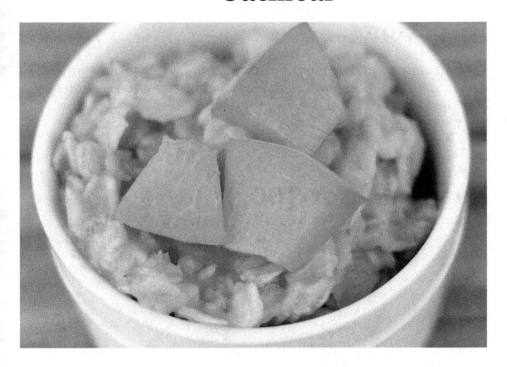

Preparation time: 10 minutes

Cooking time: 15 minutes

Servings: 4

Ingredients:

- 1 and ½ cups water

- 1 cup steel cut oats

- 1 cup orange juice

- 2 tablespoons apricots, dried and chopped 2 tablespoons coconut sugar

89

- 2 tablespoons pecans, chopped

- ¼ teaspoon cinnamon powder

Directions:

1. In a small pot, combine the oats with the water, orange juice, apricots, sugar, cinnamon and pecans, stir, bring to a simmer over medium heat, cook for 15 minutes, divide into bowls and serve for breakfast.

Enjoy!

Nutrition (for 100g):
Calories 190, Fat 3, Fiber 6, Carbs 8, Protein 5

42. Cinnamon Pear Oatmeal

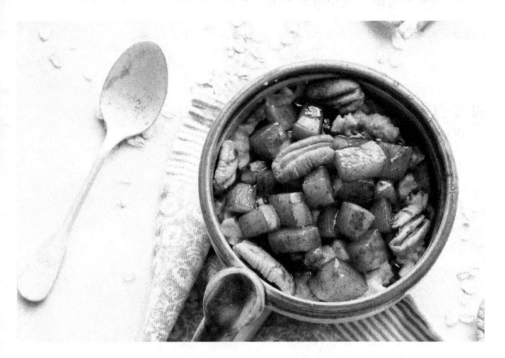

Preparation time: 10 minutes

Cooking time: 15 minutes

Servings: 3

Ingredients:

- 3 cups water

- 1 cup steel cut oats

- 1 tablespoon cinnamon powder

- 1 cup pear, cored, peeled and cubed

Directions:

1. In a small pot, combine the water with the oats, cinnamon and pear, toss, bring to a simmer over medium heat, cook for 15

minutes, divide into bowls and serve for breakfast.

Enjoy!

Nutrition (for 100g):
Calories 171, Fat 2, Fiber 5, Carbs 11, Protein 6

43. **Banana And Walnuts Bowls**

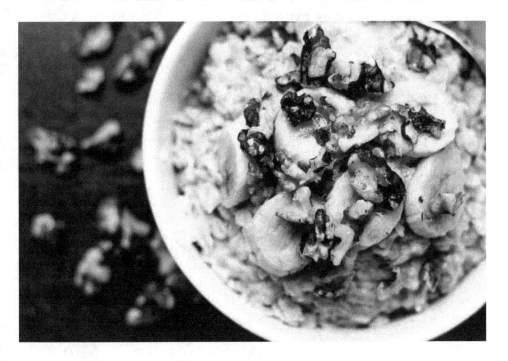

Preparation time: 10 minutes

Cooking time: 15 minutes

Servings: 4

Ingredients:

- 2 cups water

- 1 cup steel cut oats

- 1 cup almond milk

- ¼ cup walnuts, chopped

- 2 tablespoons chia seeds

- 2 bananas, peeled and mashed

- 1 teaspoon vanilla extract

Directions:

1. In a small pot, combine the water with the oats, milk, walnuts, chia seeds, bananas and vanilla, toss, bring to a simmer over medium heat, cook for 15 minutes, divide into bowls and serve for breakfast.

Enjoy!

Nutrition (for 100g):
Calories 162, Fat 4, Fiber 6, Carbs 11, Protein 4

44. Parsley Omelet

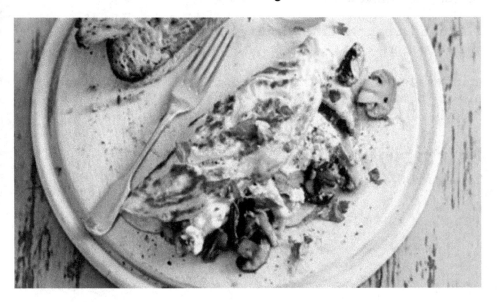

Preparation time: 10 minutes

Cooking time: 6 minutes

Servings: 6

Ingredients:

- 2 tablespoons almond milk

- A pinch of black pepper

- 6 eggs, whisked

- 2 tablespoons parsley, chopped

- 1 tablespoon low-Fat cheddar cheese, shredded 2 teaspoons olive oil

Directions:

1. In a bowl, mix the eggs with the milk, black pepper, parsley and cheese and whisk well.

2. Heat up a pan with the oil over medium-high heat, add the eggs mix, spread into the pan, cook for 3 minutes, flip, cook for 3

minutes more, divide between plates and serve for breakfast.

Enjoy!

Nutrition (for 100g):

Calories 200, Fat 4, Fiber 6, carb 13, Protein 9

45.   Cheddar Baked Eggs

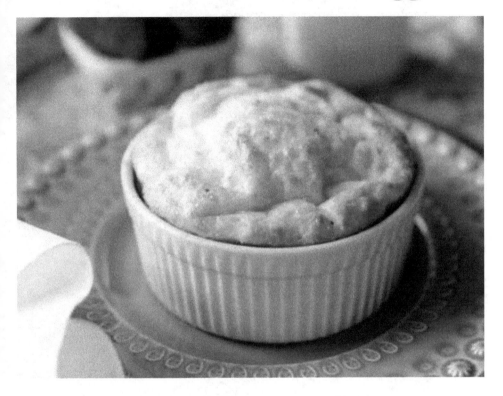

Preparation time: 10 minutes

Cooking time: 15 minutes

Servings: 4

Ingredients:

- 4 eggs

- 4 slices low-Fat cheddar

- 2 spring onions, chopped

- 1 tablespoon olive oil

- A pinch of black pepper

- 1 tablespoon cilantro, chopped

Directions:

1. Grease 4 ramekins with the oil, sprinkle green onions in each, crack an egg in each ramekins and top with cilantro and cheddar cheese.

2. Introduce in the oven and bake at 375 degrees F for 15 minutes.

3. Serve for breakfast.

Enjoy!

Nutrition (for 100g):
Calories 199, Fat 3, Fiber 7, Carbs 11, Protein 5

46. Hash Brown Mix

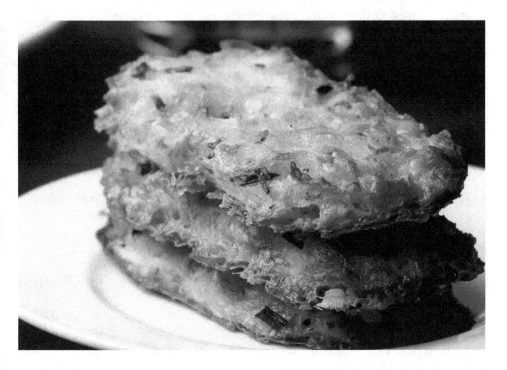

Preparation time: 10 minutes

Cooking time: 30 minutes

Servings: 6

Ingredients:

- Cooking spray

- 6 eggs

- 2 cups hash browns

- ¼ cup non-Fat milk

- ½ cup Fat-free cheddar cheese, shredded

- 1 small yellow onion, chopped

- A pinch of black pepper

- ½ green bell pepper, chopped

- ½ red bell pepper, chopped

Directions:

1. Heat up a pan greased with cooking spray over medium-high heat, add onions, green and red bell pepper, stir and cook for 4-5

minutes.

2. Add hash browns and black pepper, stir and cook for 5 minutes more.

3. In a bowl, combine the eggs with milk and cheese, whisk well, pour over the mix from the pan, introduce in the oven and bake at 380 degrees F for 20 minutes.

4. Slice, divide between plates and serve.

Enjoy!

Nutrition (for 100g):
Calories 221, Fat 4, Fiber 5, Carbs 14, Protein 6

47. Peaches Mix

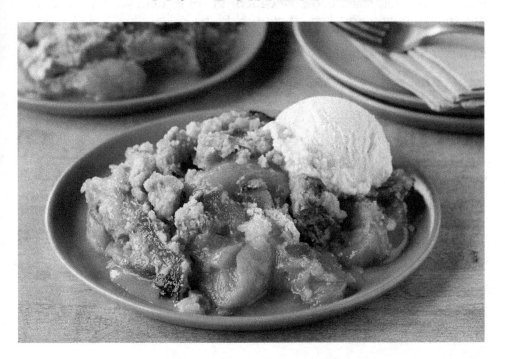

Preparation time: 10 minutes

Cooking time: 5 minutes

Servings: 4

Ingredients:

- 6 small peaches, cored and cut into wedges ¼ cup coconut sugar

- 2 tablespoons non-Fat butter

- ¼ teaspoon almond extract

Directions:

1. In a small pan, combine the peaches with sugar, butter and almond extract, toss, cook over medium-high heat for 5 minutes, divide into bowls and serve for breakfast.

Enjoy!

Nutrition (for 100g):
Calories 198, Fat 2, Fiber 6, Carbs 11, Protein 8

48. **Cinnamon Brown Rice Pudding**

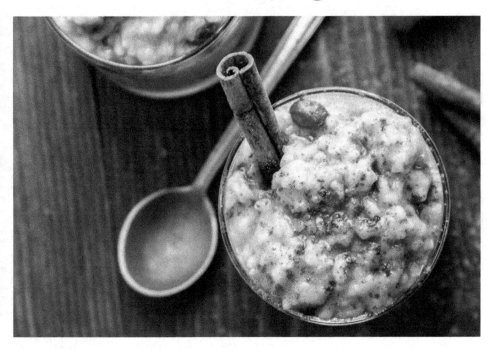

Preparation time: 10 minutes

Cooking time: 25 minutes

Servings: 4

Ingredients:

- 1 cup brown rice

- 1 and ½ cups water

- 1 tablespoon vanilla extract

- 1 tablespoon cinnamon powder

- 1 tablespoon non-Fat butter

- ½ cup coconut cream, unsweetened

Directions:

1. In a pot, combine the rice with the water, vanilla, cinnamon, butter and cream, stir, bring to a simmer over medium heat, cook for 25 minutes, divide into bowls and serve for breakfast.

Enjoy!

Nutrition (for 100g):
Calories 182, Fat 4, Fiber 7, Carbs 11, Protein 6

49. **Cream Basmati Rice Pudding**

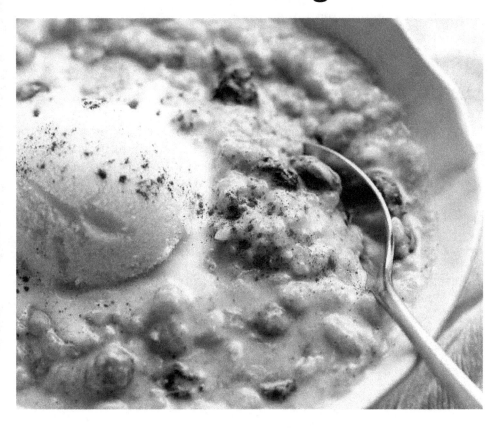

Preparation time: 10 minutes

Cooking time: 25 minutes

Servings: 6

Ingredients:

- 2 cups coconut milk
- 1 and ¼ cups water

- 1 cup basmati rice

- 2 tablespoons coconut sugar

- ¾ cup coconut cream

- 1 teaspoon vanilla extract

Directions:

1. In a pot, combine the coconut milk with the water, rice, sugar, cream and vanilla, toss, bring to a simmer over medium heat, cook for 25 minutes, stirring often, divide into bowls and serve for breakfast.

Enjoy!

Nutrition (for 100g):
Calories 191, Fat 4, Fiber 7, Carbs 11, Protein 6

50. Zucchini And Sweet Potato Bowl

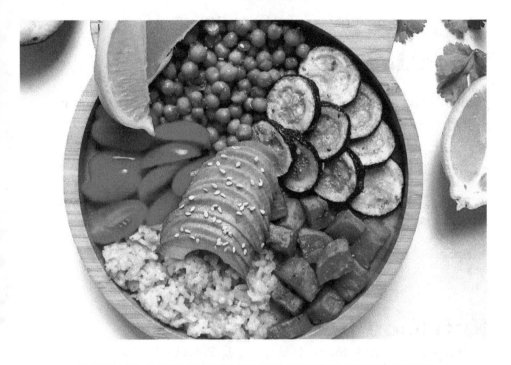

Preparation time: 10 minutes

Cooking time: 10 minutes

Servings: 2

Ingredients:

- 1 big zucchini, cut with the spiralizer

- Salt and black pepper to the taste

- ¼ cup extra virgin olive oil

- ½ avocado, peeled, pitted and cubed

- 2 tablespoons green onions, chopped

- 2 garlic cloves, chopped

- 2 sweet potatoes, peeled and cubed

Directions:

1. Heat up a pan with half of the olive oil over medium-high heat, add potatoes, stir and cook for 8 minutes.

2. In your food processor, mix avocado with the rest of the oil, garlic, salt and pepper and blend well.

3. Put zucchini noodles in a bowl, add avocado cream and sweet potatoes and toss to coat.

4. Sprinkle green onions and serve for breakfast.

Enjoy!

Nutrition (for 100g):
Calories 171, Fat 3, Fiber 3, Carbs 11, Protein 4

Conclusion

Thank you for reading this cookbook. In general, breakfast is going to consist of protein and whole grains. A lot of people are under the impression that they need to go for protein bars as their breakfast but this really isn't true. Instead look at your cooking ingredients as possible sources for a Dash Diet Breakfast meal. Eggs are an excellent source of protein and can be eaten boiled or scrambled with added vegetables such as spinach or broccoli. You could even add some turkey bacon to the mix.

For breakfast you should drink a Dash Diet Juice for fruit juice or a cup of tea or coffee with skimmed milk. Do not have any soda or fruit juice containing added sugar as they can cause blood sugar spikes that will make you feel more hungry. This is one of the main reasons why so many people struggle with weight loss – because they're not getting the right foods that break down slowly and even help to fill up your stomach if it's rumbling. If you do need something to sweeten your tea, go for an artificial sweetener such as sucralose instead of sugar, honey or fructose.

Always go with water or unsweetened tea. You should never have soda, as it's loaded with sugar and high fructose corn syrup which leads to insulin spikes. It makes you hungrier and you're going to crave more sugary foods throughout the day. Water is always the way to go for a healthy breakfast, it keeps your metabolism working correctly as well as keeping your energy levels up. If you need another kick in the morning, try a cup of green tea rather than black tea – studies show that green tea actually increases your metabolism by 4%.

The tips for Dash Diet are the same as any other diet that you try out. Make sure you're getting enough sleep, so your body is ready to take in the nutrients. Always read everything in your breakfast before you eat it, as many pre-packaged breakfasts often contain large amounts of sugar or salt, which will slow down weight loss. I hope you liked this!